Dear Child of God,

"But even the very hairs of your all numbered. Fear not therefore: ye are of more value than many sparrows."

Blessings!
Claudia Hamilton

Curly Girls, Love Your Curls!

Curly Girls, Love Your Curls!

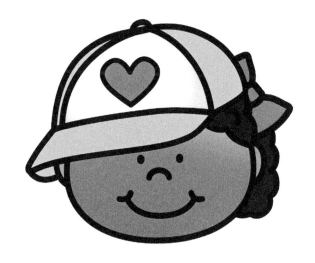

Claudia M. Hamilton

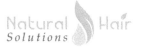

Interior Art Credit: Laura Strickland and Krista Wallden

Scripture taken from the King James Version of the Bible.

WestBow Press books may be ordered through booksellers or by contacting:

WestBow Press
A Division of Thomas Nelson & Zondervan
1663 Liberty Drive
Bloomington, IN 47403
www.westbowpress.com
1 (866) 928-1240

ISBN: 978-1-5127-8615-6 (sc)
ISBN: 978-1-5127-8616-3 (e)

Library of Congress Control Number: 2017906880

Print information available on the last page.

WestBow Press rev. date: 5/3/2017

A Note from the Author

I trust that you will enjoy learning how to take care of your lovely tresses! Never be ashamed of your gorgeous curls. God gave them to you because you are truly unique☺. Oh, and by the way, don't forget to expand your vocabulary along the way...you'll see what I'm talking about as you read this fabulous and informative story about your curls. Enjoy the journey!

If you ever wish to communicate with me regarding your crowning glory, ask your parents to send me an email at restoringyournaturalhairitage@gmail.com.

God Bless You,

Claudia M. Hamilton

"But if a woman have long hair, it is a glory to her: for her hair is given her for a covering". I Corinthians 11:15 KJV

Hi! My name is Curly Girl. Can you guess why everyone calls me Curly Girl? That's right!

I HAVE CURLY HAIR.

I used to be soooooo embarrassed about my curly hair, until the day my mom and dad sat me down and explained why curls make me so unique.

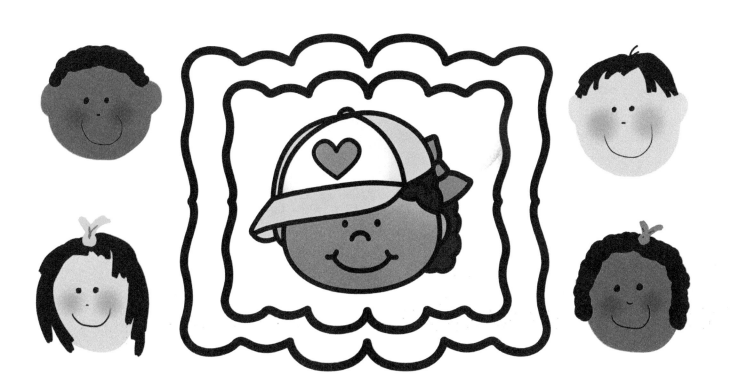

I'm one of a kind...made in the image of God! My curls are just like thumbprints. There's no other curly girl in the world with curls quite like mine.

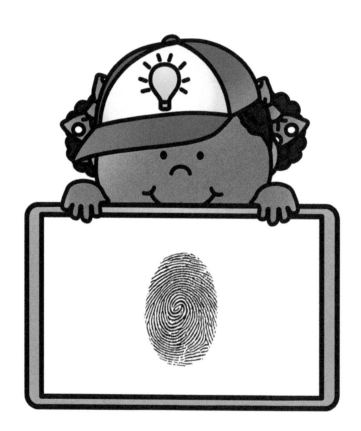

Curls come in different shapes, colours and sizes...they range from wavy to tightly coiled. I'd say that my curls are somewhere in between.

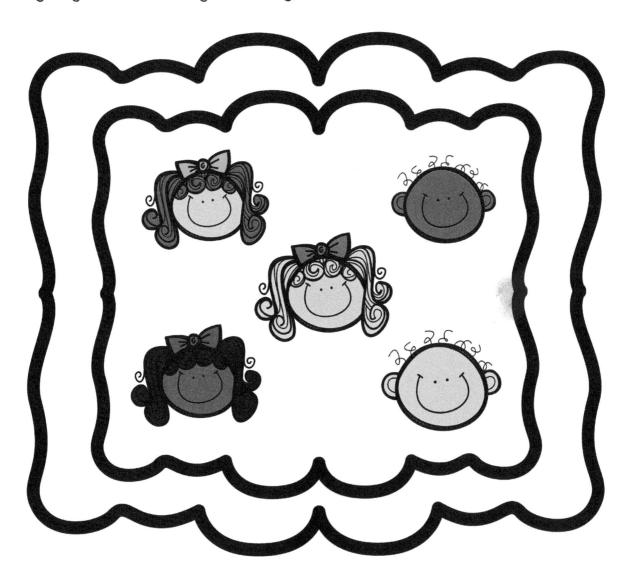

The coolest thing about having curls is that I can straighten them with a hair dryer or flat iron (as long as I use a heat protectant so that my beautiful curls will never lose their bounce and definition when I'm ready to rock my curls again!). Did I hear you say versatile? That's a pretty sophisticated word. Look it up in the dictionary and try to use it: V-E-R-S-A-T-I-L-E

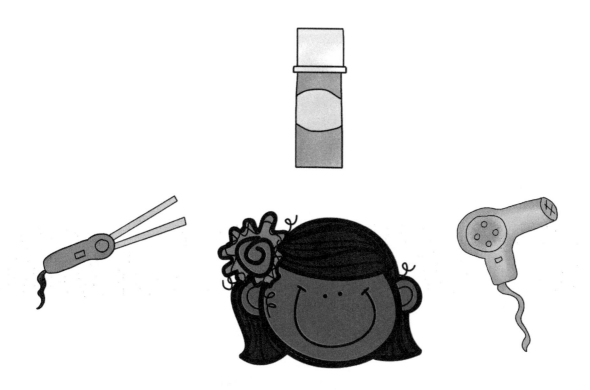

It has a nice ring to it, doesn't it? Yes, my curls are versatile.

My mom says that when she was a kid, she was sooooo embarrassed about her curls and worst of all, she wondered why her hair never grew past the nape of her neck. While, most of her friends had long flowing hair that they styled with ribbons and fancy hair bands, mom's never seemed to look quite right when she wore those hair accessories. She tried her best to control those tight coils, but NOTHING ever seemed to work!

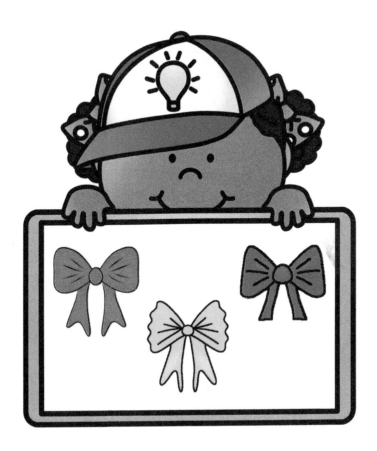

After many years of trying leave-in conditioners and hair-growth serums, mom still could not successfully grow her hair!!!! She began to wonder, "Why not????" Her mommy didn't know, her daddy didn't know and neither did her aunts and uncles. This was a mystery that she was determined to solve.

There's another sophisticated word that you should look up in the dictionary:

D-E-T-E-R-M-I-N-E-D

Finally, just before my mom's 40ᵗʰ birthday, she went on a mission to find out why her hair just would not grow. Mom decided to expand her career as a teacher and she became a certified HAIR PRACTITIONER, so that she could teach all the curly girls in the world how to take care of their hair. Hair Practitioners can help you take care of your hair and scalp problems. They can use a derma-scope to check the condition of your scalp, so that they can tell you what to use to keep your scalp healthy and to make your curls the best curls ever!

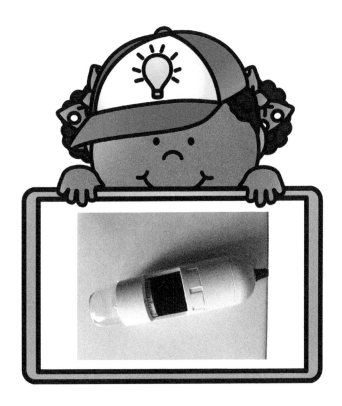

Now, instead of teaching in the classroom, my mom teaches ladies how to make their tresses one-of-a-kind and truly unique...but you know what my mom really wants to be, even more than a Teacher and a Hair Practitioner? She wants to become a Trichologist, because she wants to help ALL the women in the world feel good about their hair, whether curly or straight, long or short! She wants to diagnose and provide treatment for all scalp diseases.

T-R-I-C-H-O-L-O-G-I-S-T...I think you should check the internet for that definition.

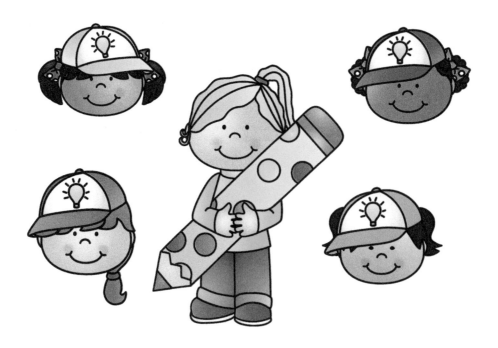

Since my mom knows so much about hair, I ask her many questions to make sure that I am taking the best care of my hair. I've learned that it is important to keep my hair clean. Washing my hair often, is a very good habit, even while I am wearing braids, twists or extensions.

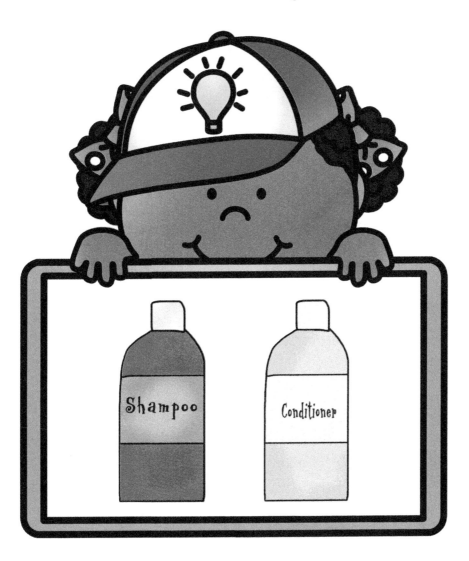

While washing my hair, I never swirl it around in too many directions because that just causes too many tangles. Instead, I use a special technique to keep my hair de-tangled while washing...It's as easy as 1-2-3!

1. I divide my hair in four to six sections (using a tail comb).
2. I use a spray bottle to spritz my hair with water then I apply a silicone-free conditioner to each section and de-tangle with my fingers.
3. I twist each conditioned section then tuck them away in Bantu knots.

When I finish detangling my hair, I rinse each section with warm water, gently stroking my hair downward from the root toward the ends. I stroke from root to ends to make sure that the cuticle layer of each strand lays flat so that the moisture stays in and my hair strands don't stick together like Velcro. The cuticle layer of my hair is the protective layer that keeps my strands strong. If I swirl my hair in too many directions, the cuticles will stick up and eventually break off.

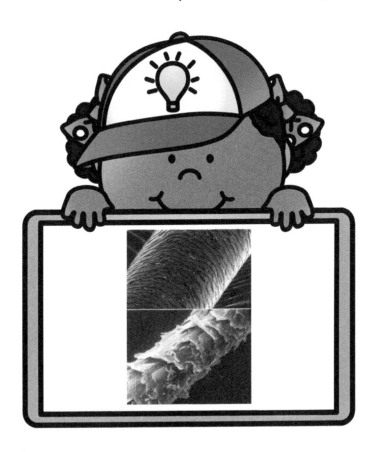

After I finish rinsing my hair, I use a sulfate-free shampoo and wash each section of my hair one-by-one (always remembering to scrub my scalp with the pads of my fingers and not my fingernails). Then I rinse my hair with warm water. I add more silicone-free conditioner to each section and I rinse with lukewarm water. I use a microfiber towel to pat my hair dry and sometimes I wrap my head with a cotton t-shirt to absorb the water.

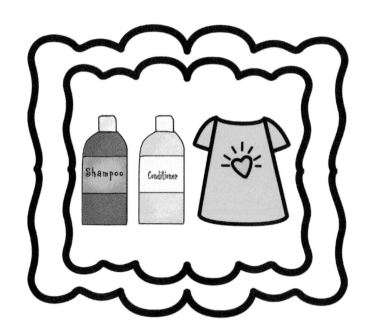

Can you find the word, A-B-S-O-R-B in the dictionary? What does it mean?

I lightly spritz my hair with distilled water before applying a natural leave-in conditioner and a Shea Butter sealant. The water opens my cuticles, the leave-in conditioner softens my hair and the Shea Butter seals the moisture in my hair for a few days. I try not to use products containing: mineral oil, petroleum and silicone, so that my hair will stay nice and soft for as long as possible. I don't EVER want my hair to get dry and brittle or else my strands will break into a million little pieces on the floor. I want my hair to stay on my head where hair belongs.

I **never** use a fine-toothed comb to de-tangle my hair because I don't want my hair to break. I **always** use a wide-toothed shampoo comb (starting from ends to root) to gently remove knots and tangles, then I braid or twist my hair so that the next day when I undo my hair I have the best curls ever. It's so easy to take care of my beautiful curls!

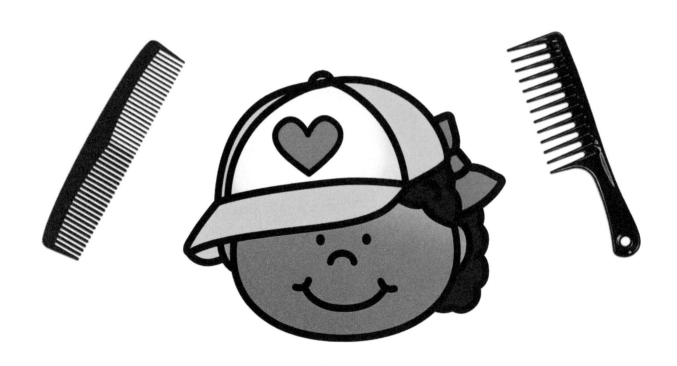

CPSIA information can be obtained
at www.ICGtesting.com
Printed in the USA
LVOW05s1929231017
553500LV00022B/163/P